Hidden Truth
of Cancer

Keiichi Morishita, M. D.

translated by
Herman Aihara

George Ohsawa Macrobiotic Foundation
Chico, California

Editing by Kathy Keller
Cover design by Carl Campbell
Text layout and design by Carl Ferré

First Edition   1976
Current Edition, edited and reformated   2010 Jan 10

© copyright 1976 by
George Ohsawa Macrobiotic Foundation
    PO Box 3998, Chico, California 95927-3998
    530-566-9765; fax 530-566-9768
    www.ohsawamacrobiotics.com; gomf@ohsawamacrobiotics.com

Published with the help of East West Center for Macrobiotics
    www.eastwestmacrobiotics.com

ISBN 978-0-918860-25-5

Contents

Translator's note: The correct translation of "red blood cell" from Japanese is "red globule." However, I have used the phrase "blood cell" instead of "globule" in order to avoid confusion for the reader. The reader should also be advised that a blood cell is different from a regular (body) cell in its structure and property. The red blood cell is especially different from the regular (body or tissue) cell in that it usually does not contain a nucleus, whereas a white blood cell contains a nucleus.

Introduction

The contemporary life sciences, especially biology and medicine, have now reached a turning point. Some scientists say, "The revolution of the life sciences will occur in the last half of the 20th Century along with historical research and thought about the progress of natural science." I agree with this opinion.

However, modern medicine has many paradoxes and dogmas in its theories. These paradoxes are mostly due to the acceptance of the basic concepts of German physicist Virchow's theory *Omnis cellula e cellula,* that is, all cells come only from cells. This has been generally believed to be a "golden rule" in the biological and medical sciences.

Science is a study of the relationship between cause and effect in the phenomena of nature. However, Virchow's concept prohibits further thinking regarding the cause or the origin of the cell. Medical science will never develop or progress from this concept. It is a cancerous theory. This unscientific theory has caused many superstitions in the medical field.

Cancer is one example of such superstitions. If we know the cause and mechanism of cancer, we need not fear it. Modern science is afraid of cancer, just as primitives are afraid of an electric light. The real cancer is not in our bodies but in the mentality of the scientist who rigidly believes that all cells arise from other cells.

The problem of cancer in our civilization is beneficial because it will bring forth a revolution in modern medicine. If modern medicine does not change its direction, cancer will become a fatal disease, not only for men, but for modern medicine which has spread its malignant effects on the whole of society. Therefore, cancer in this century has a historical mission: to correct modern medicine.

Modern medicine will never end the disaster of cancer, which is criminally condemned and becomes explosive when handled violently. However, it is a faithful servant if we handle it gently, knowing its character. I am trying here to write the truth about cancer from the historical and macroscopic viewpoint so that you may understand that cancer is not our enemy but our benefactor, because it teaches us how to live healthfully and happily.

Chapter One

The Basic Problem of Cancer

According to modern medicine, the definition of cancer is: *malignant cells that suddenly mutate from normal cells, for some reason, and are manifested by reduced control over growth and function, leading to serious adverse effects on the host through invasive growth and metastasis.*

Several questions arise from this definition of cancer. First, why have such cells formed? If we can answer these questions, we can cure or prevent cancer. Medical scholars all over the world have researched these questions, ardently, for over a half century. Unfortunately, we have not yet received adequate answers from them. This is due, neither to the insufficient efforts of the scientists nor to the shortage of financial support for research. It is due to the ideas or beliefs existing in the mentality of the scientists who conduct cancer research. In other words, their ideas or concepts of "What is Life?" "What is a cell?" "What is the origin of a cell?" "How does a cell grow?" are incorrect. I regret that all scientists are searching for a cause of cancer in the wrong direction, and therefore, their effort will be in vain.

The above definition of cancer was proposed by the disciples of Virchow who blindly accepted his doctrine *Omnis cellula e cellula,* i.e., all cells come only from cells. Since this theory is completely incorrect, this definition doesn't correspond with reality and lacks scientific thinking. For example, "for some reason" is an expression admitting ignorance of the reason. Therefore, this is not a definition of cancer.

"Suddenly" is another expression of ignorance. If we know the cause, we can anticipate the effect. Solving the problem of cancer using such a definition is like looking for fish in the trees.

We are told that one-third to one-half of all cancer could be cured if patients would see a specialist for prompt treatment in the early stages. However, what the early stage is, is not clear. Could this be an excuse of the doctors who can't cure cancer?

There are three treatments for cancer in Western medicine:

1. Surgery
2. Chemical treatment
3. Radiation treatment

1. Surgery: Surgery is based on the idea that the removal of the symptoms is a cure. They are committing two errors with this idea. First, cancerous symptoms (cells) are the result not the cause, therefore elimination of cancerous cells will not cure cancer. It is a temporary cure. Second, any disease, including cancer, is a sickness of the whole body. Therefore, removal of cancerous cells on one part of the body will cause growth of cancerous cells on another. I would say that if cancer can be cured by surgery it can be more easily cured without it because the operation weakens the body against resistence to cancer.

2. Chemical treatment: There are several anti-cancerous drugs. I doubt their efficacy. The idea of "anti-cancer" is disagreeable to me. Since cancerous cells are part of our body, the destruction of such cells, by drugs, will inevitably destroy our normal cells. Therefore, medicine must find a drug which will strengthen our normal cells, which will control the cancerous cells and prevent their growth and function. In other words, not an antidrug but a complementary drug.

3. Radiation treatment: This is a most dangerous treatment: radiation has been an important cancer producing factor since 1902. The cancerous cell will be destroyed by the radiation, but the normal cells will be mutated to cancer cells by the exposed weak radiation. Thus, there is little evidence to confirm the claim that prompt treatment of cancer in the early stages will cure most cases. Often, early treatment leads to early death. There must exist many cases where cancer was cured naturally, without serious medication, when the early symptoms were not noticed.

Medical science believes that cancer is incurable (another name for death). A diagnosis of cancer means a death sentence. This is nothing but a proof of the incompetence of modern medicine. However, cancer is not such an incurable, deadly disease.

Medical doctors often say that it was not cancer to begin with when they see someone who was cured of cancer after being abandoned by medical doctors. This is a doctor's excuse. In reality, cancer can be more readily cured if we avoid wrong medication. At least we may live longer if we avoid wrong medications. Dr. John Cryle showed many cases in which cancer patients survived many years without medication. In cancerous experimental animals there are some deaths, but some cure themselves naturally. These animals had been fed refined foods. Therefore, their resistance to cancer must be weak. In such animals, cancer will be produced without inoculation. However, we can change the cancer production rate by changing the quality and the quantity of foods. For example, a mouse who produces 70% cancerous cells 1-2 years after birth can reduce this rate to almost zero simply by reducing its food 1/3 to 1/5.

In my experiments, I fed mixed grains and salt to chickens who were suffering from leukemia. The chickens were cured completely from their cancer. This result revealed that a close relationship between cancer and nutrition exists.

However, the "real" nutrition cannot be encompassed by the three main aliments: carbohydrates, proteins, and fats, nor by caloric intake.

Recently, many animals in zoos have died from cancer. For example, sea lions have died from cancer of the urethra and monkeys have died from cancer of the esophagus. Their intake of domestic food must be related to this fact because they never die from cancer when they select foods from their own natural habitats.

To confirm this, there is an interesting experiment made by Dr. Robert McCarrison, the chief physician of the Indian Nutritional Institute. He gave the Hunza diet to a group of 1,000 healthy mice, then he gave the Indian diet to another group of 2,000 healthy mice. After 27 months, he made autopsies and pathologically compared the two groups. The results were astonishing. The mice which were fed the Hunza diet were completely healthy. There were no signs of sickness among them. However, most of the mice which were fed the Indian diet showed symptoms of many sicknesses such as eye impairment, tumors, tooth decay, stunted growth, falling hair, anemia, skin, heart, kidney, stomach and intestinal diseases.

When he gave the English diet to the final group of 1,000 mice, they not only showed the above symptoms, but also impairment of the nervous system. They became so cruel that they bit one another.

Here are the diets given to the three groups of mice:

1. Hunza diet—chapati (a bread made from whole grains), soy bean malt, raw carrot, raw cabbage and raw milk (without pasteurization).
2. Indian diet—rice (white), beans, cooked vegetables with spices (which Indians eat daily).
3. English diet—white bread, margarine, tea with sugar, cooked vegetables, canned meat, jam and jello.

This experiment reveals much concerning diet, not only for animals, but also for man. It shows us that longevity of race, character of race and the cause of disease is dependent on diet. Food is life. My new blood theory, which I will make a report on later, will show the relationship between food and life. If modern civilization continues as it has, all civilized countries will be destroyed completely, not by war, but by diseases such as cancer, heart or mental disease. During the present critical period, only the continued existence of Hunza Land offers hope for the future. Hunza Land has remained isolated from other countries during the last 2,000 years. It never suffered from plague, such as leprosy in the 14th Century, pestilence in the 15th Century, syphilis in the 16th Century, smallpox in the 17th and 18th Centuries, and tuberculosis in the 19th Century.

The Hunza people are immune to the cancer and heart diseases of the 20th Century. They have never suffered from any disease. In this unhealthy age, this is miraculous and incredible.

The problem of cancer has no solution without giving thought to the fundamental question: Why have the people of Hunza Land been living with superior health when other peoples are suffering from so many diseases?

If we find the basic principle key to solving the cancer problem, we can apply it to all other diseases. Symptomatic medicine, not realizing the causes of cancer, can never cure it completely.

Chapter Two

Blood Physiology

All living things are divided into two categories, plant and animal. Plants are stationary; therefore, their roots can grow into the earth and receive nutrition. Animals, however, cannot be rooted because they move around. How then does an animal receive its nutrition? The intestine does the job. The intestine is the portable root of an animal.

The root of a plant picks up its nutrition from the soil in the form of inorganic matter and then transforms it to organic matter. An animal receives its nutrition from the vegetables, which have grown from the soil. Therefore, both the plant and animal are eating nutrition from the soil. From this point of view they are not essentially different.

According to modern physiology the roles of the intestine are digestion and absorption of foods. In reality, the intestine does its job more dynamically.

The villus of the intestinal wall is like an amoeba. The digested foods go into the villus, not by simple physical process, but by a biological process. In this biological process, physiological blood production takes place. In other words, the villus takes the digested food stuffs into its structure, assimilates and finally transforms them into the red blood cells.

Furthermore, these red blood cells circulate throughout the body and transform themselves into the body cells (such as liver, muscles, brain cells, etc.)

Modern medicine and biology teach that cells grow by the division of cells. For example, one liver cell will divide into two, two into four, etc. This is true only under special conditions, like in vitro (test tube). It never happens, however, in the normal living body. From my study, the red blood cells gather and form the various organs and tissues. Therefore, our body is a transformation of food. Our constitution and character depend upon our food. Food is life.

The schematic diagram of the red blood cell formation:

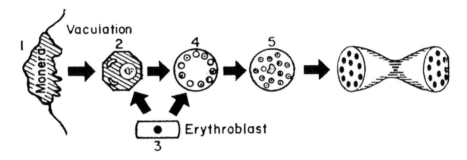

1) The food monera is surrounded by the intestine villi.

2) Formation of liquid hole inside of the monera.

3) This liquid hole changes to the villus cell.

4) This cell develops and becomes a "mother" red blood cell (erythroblast).

5) Finally, this erythroblast contains many red blood cells. The red blood cells enter the blood vessels and circulate throughout the body. What then is the function of the red blood cell?

According to modern physiology, the main role of the red blood cell is considered to be the transfer of oxygen and carbon dioxide. In other words, a red blood cell carries oxygen to a cell and carries carbon dioxide back from the cell to the blood. However, in reality it is not so simple.

The most important role of a red blood cell, which apparently is not recognized at the present time, is that the red blood cell develops into the various cell structures such as bone marrow, adipose tissue, muscular tissue, liver, spleen, kidney, brain, etc. The red blood cell is nothing but the fundamental material of our body.

The concept that a red blood cell transforms to a body cell is unique and, along with the concept of food transforming into red blood cells, has not before been imagined. Since these conceptions are new in the field of science, there will be much resistance before they are accepted by scientists. In my opinion, these concepts must be justified by the progress of science—not by the current academic opinion.

In conclusion, in our body the digested food (which is organic matter) transforms itself into the simplest life (a red blood cell), and this simple life transforms to a higher stage of life—a body cell.

According to my theory of evolution, there once existed only inorganic matter on the earth. Then the inorganic changed to organic matter, the organic matter to protein and the protein (built up) to simple life. The coordination of this simple life developed to the higher life of animal and then finally reached the stage of man.

This fantastic evolution of life is not a mere theory of anthropology. It is taking place in our body every day, every second. It has taken billions of years to evolve from the inorganic stage to man. However, in our body it takes only one or two days. What a miracle we have been doing! What a miracle our life is! Our body is a wonderful, fantastic phenomenon.

In the case of stomach illness, intestinal diarrhea, or when fasting, the intestine stops production of red blood cells. Then the *body cells* start reverse transformation to *red blood cells*. For example, diarrhea causes weight loss. The reason is that the adipose tissues transform back to red blood cells—although modern physiology explains this phenomena as the burning of adipose tissue to produce energy.

Why do body cells transform back to the red blood cells? The quantity of red blood cells in our body cannot decrease indefinitely because our body cannot function smoothly without a certain amount of red blood cells.

The number of red blood cells is about 5 million per cubic millimeter in humans. It rarely reaches less than 3 million. These cells must supply oxygen to the brain or kidney because these organs consume a great deal of oxygen. If the number of red blood cells decreases to less than 3 million, the supply of oxygen will not be enough for these organs and eventually such important organs will stop their function. Therefore, when the production of red blood cells stops, as in the case of fasting or sickness, the body cells begin to revert back to red blood cells This phenomena begins with the adipose tissue. The result is loss of weight.

Rabbits have 5.5 million to 6 million red blood cells. If they are fed nothing they will die in 2 to 3 weeks. However, the amount of red blood cells rarely decreases to less than 3 million. Why does the rabbit keep a constant amount of red blood cells without producing them physiologically? The reason is the same as in the above human case. Therefore, such a rabbit shows empty body cells after autopsy. For example, the liver will retain its shape but its cytoplasm will have diminished. The cells of all organs of the rabbit (dead from starving) reveal considerable damage. The cells of the liver, kidney and even the brain become porous. This is caused, as I stated before, by reverse transformation. Through this reverse transformation, our body organs can function with a minimum amount of red blood cells until the very end of life.

Modern medicine distinguishes between the red blood cells and the tissue (body) cell. In reality, however, they are related to each other and can be transformed (one into the other) in both directions. When a person is healthy, the red blood cells change to body cells; when one is sick, the reverse will happen.

Modern physiology believes that bone marrow produces blood. In 1952 four physiologists, Drs. Donn, Cunningham, Sabin, and Jordan performed a two-week starvation experiment using chickens and doves. They found that the red blood cells had been produced from bone marrow. This experiment is the basic proof of that theory. This experiment will be explained clearly by my theory. When fasting the cells of the bone marrow, adipose tissue, muscular tissue, liver, etc. transform to red blood cells in a certain order. The process begins with the bone marrow. Therefore, in spite of what the four physiologists thought, this is not normal blood production. It is a compensatory blood production. The normal physiological blood production is done by the intestine.

The Danger of Radiation

The most important phenomena with regard to the results of radiation are leukemia and unrecoverable malignant anemia. Leukemia, especially, is the most characteristic product of radiation. Leukemia is evidenced not only in the atomic radiation sufferers in Hiroshima and Nagasaki, but also in increasing numbers of infants and babies whose mothers received a great deal of radiation during pregnancy.

Here I will discuss the cause of leukemia and anemia caused by radiation.

Leukemia is a sickness which results in the malignant increase of white blood cells. Its mechanism is not clear to modern science.

Since scientists believe the theory that blood is produced by the bone marrow, they are searching for the root of this sickness within the bone marrow. Since the blood, however, is never produced in the bone marrow under normal physiological conditions, their effort will not bring any satisfactory results.

Under normal physiological conditions, the intestine produces the blood. In other words, the digested food moneras transform to red blood cells in the intestine villi. These red blood cells not only carry oxygen to the body cells and carry back waste carbon dioxide from the body cells, but also have the important function of transforming themselves into body cells.

The gathered red blood cells transform into the kinds of cells which they are contacting while passing through the intermediate white blood cell stage.

Dr. Chishima and I call this phenomena the differentiation of the red blood cells. Our body cells do not grow by cell division but by the transformation of the red blood cells. Therefore, the basic material of all organs, tissue, and fat is the red blood cell. Sometimes in this process, the intermediate stage of the transformation—the white blood cell—is not clearly observed.

When we are sick or physiologically abnormal or under conditions of stress—as in the case of an operation, fasting, chronic diarrhea, neurosis, etc.—the production of blood in the intestine stops and the body cells transform reversely to the red blood cells in order to keep constant the amount of red blood cells. This is possible because all body cells were produced from red blood cells originally. Thus, between the red blood cells and the body cells there is this reversible relationship.

Why does this reverse transformation (from body cell to red blood cell) happen?

Our blood stream must keep constant the amount of red blood cells in order to supply enough oxygen to the important organs such as the brain or kidneys, which cannot live even a few minutes without oxygen. Therefore, this reverse transformation compensates for the emergency created by the diminishing production of red blood cells. In such cases, bone marrow, adipose tissue, and muscular tissue transform to red blood cells first because these are cells of secondary importance compared with other body cells. The modern theory of blood production in the bone marrow is the result of the misunderstanding of this compensatory phenomenon.

Now we are going to consider the cause of leukemia and unrecoverable malignant anemia by the Chishima-Morishita theory.

The stomach and intestines are the most sensitive organs in our body. A little sentimental upset has a big influence on the stomach or intestine, and will sometimes cause an ulcer in those organs. Therefore, it is easy to imagine that radiation will have a strong effect on the stomach or the intestine. It was revealed from the patients who died in the Pierre Curie Hospital that the damage to the stomach and intestines was most apparent.

In Japan, in the case of atomic radiation sufferers or radiotherapy patients who had been neglected, damage to the stomach and intestines has been noticed more and more.

Unrecoverable malignant anemia is the result of severe damage to the intestinal villi which causes the intestine to stop its function of blood formation. This disease often happens when a great amount of radiation has been applied to a patient. The term "unrecoverable" indicates that recovery will not occur as long as the doctors search the bone marrow for the cause.

What is the cause of leukemia?

In the case of radiation leukemia not only the stomach or intestines but also many other body cells will have been damaged or retarded. As a result, the red blood cells are no longer able to transform to body cells because this transformation needs strong guidance from the body cells in order to proceed. When the body cells are damaged or retarded by radiation, they lose guiding power which is necessary for the red blood cells to transform to body cells. Instead, the red blood cells remain in the Intermediate state—white blood cells. [Translator's note: Please try to explain the above theory by Yin and Yang.]

Blood Formation and the Red Blood Cell

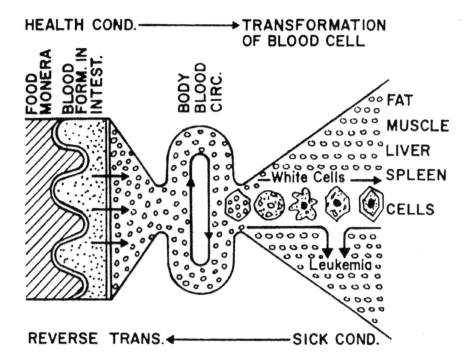

There is another reason for the increase in white blood cells in radiation leukemia. In the case of diminishing blood formation by the intestines, the body cells will normally transform back to red blood cells. However, the retarded body cells cannot complete their transformation to the red blood cells and remain in the intermediate stage of white blood cells.

In short, there are two reasons for the occurrence of excess white blood cells in the case of radiation damage.

1. The ability of transformation in the red blood cells is weakened and/or the *guiding* power of the body cells is weakened. This affects the power of the body cells to assimilate and lead the red blood cells to transform to the same kind of body cells when they come into contact with each other.

2. When the intestines stop their function of producing red blood cells, the body cells start reverse transformation and produce red blood cells under normal conditions. However, if the body cells are damaged, this transformation will not be completed, and the cells will stay in the intermediate stage (white blood cells) between the body cells and the red blood cells.

From these two physiological reasons, the white blood cells increase.

Red Blood Cells ⇄ White Blood Cells ⇄ Body Cells

Thus, the cause and mechanism of leukemia can be clearly understood by our theory. It is a stage of increased intermediate cells between the red blood cell and the body cell stages.

Chapter Three

The Origin of the Cancer Cell and its Character

The belief in Virchow's concept that a "cell comes only from another cell" is the major obstacle to a study of the true origin of the cancer cell. If this theory is true, a cancer cell must come from another cancer cell. As a result of this thinking, three theories have been proposed concerning the origin of cancer cells:

1. A cancer cell has intruded from the outside. There is no solid evidence for this hypothesis, and it has therefore been neglected even by those who believe in the Virchow theory.

2. A cancer cell has existed with the body from the embryonic stage. According to Dr. Cohnheim, the origin of cancer is the intrusion of certain cells of the embryo into another part of the body, thus causing abnormal growth. This hypothesis also has not received much support.

3. The sudden mutation of normal cells to cancer cells. This theory is the most accepted by those in modern medicine. However, it cannot explain the mechanism of the mutation from a normal cell to a cancer cell. Hence, the use of the word "sudden." The concept of sudden mutation is a refuge by which Virchow's concept (a cell comes only from another cell) can survive. As I said before, science is research into the law of relationship existing between cause and result. The concept of sudden mutation is an expression that one has

given up his scientific intention, because "sudden" is another word for "unknown reason," "at random" or "without any reasonable, definable cause." Therefore, the words "sudden mutation" must be thrown into the waste basket if one is to try to be honest with his scientific theory.

The Mechanism of Cancer Cell Growth

What is the cause of the sudden mutation from normal cells to malignant cells? This is the next problem with which orthodox medicine is faced. Generally speaking, in modern medicine there are three factors for such causes:

1. Chemical factors—tar, coloring chemicals, etc.

2. Physical factors—radiation

3. Biological factors—cancer virus (viruses)

1. Chemical factors: It has been noticed that within certain professions there is a tendency toward cancer. For example, laborers who handle coal-tar often develop cancer on their hands or sexual organs. Therefore, tar has been considered a carcinogen. Professor Yamakiwa experimented with this. He spread tar on the skin of rabbits for two years. The rabbits developed a cancer. However, the cancer did not develop in exactly the same spot where the tar was spread, but in its surrounding area. He did not explain the reason. This question must be clarified in order to approve of this theory. In my opinion, the cancer was caused by "tar and physiological conditions."

"Cigarette smoking is the cause of lung cancer." This is the same kind of concept. "Death caused by lung cancer," stated WHO (World Health Organization) in its September 1965 report, "is increasing every year." It has doubled in 10 years in Europe. Death rate by lung cancer is six times greater in men than women. This considers smoking a more important factor than air pollution because men are heavier smokers than women. Cigarette smoking may be a factor in lung cancer, but it would be one-sided to consider smoking as the cause of cancer.

In an animal experiment, one can produce skin cancer by spreading tar on the skin. However, my experiment revealed that when the test animals were fed animal fat (especially cholesterol), this tendency increased. WHO's report should have also taken the diet into consideration.

The death rate by lung cancer doubled in ten years, but the consumption of cigarettes may not have doubled. If people increase the consumption of animal fat or protein in their diet, the death rate will increase more than double...even if the amount of smoking remains the same.

In conclusion, I believe that the increased death rate must have a close relationship with increased consumption of animal foods. This is a greater factor than smoking.

Modern scientists tend to consider only the factors existing outside of and neglect the factors existing within our body. The most important determinant of such factors within is our food. Modern industrialized and commercialized foods contain many poisons or carcinogens. Please read *Poisons in Your Foods* by William Longgood or *Silent Spring* by Rachel Carson. Even drugs sometimes cause cancer. For example, nitrogen mustard has been used as an anti-cancer drug but it has also had the effect of causing cancer.

2. Physical factors: A report has stated that a patient treated with x-ray radiation for a rash, developed cancer in the exact location where the radiation had been given. In this case, the cancer appeared on the legs and amputation was necessary. What a tragedy! Cancer or leukemia cases among newborn babies have been increasing re-

cently. This situation may be caused by the mother receiving x-ray examinations too often during her pregnancy.

There are other factors such as ultraviolet radiation, heat, injury, etc. which may cause cancer. However, physical, physiological condition and diet are the most important factors. Cancer seldom occurs in persons whose bodies are functioning properly.

3. Biological factors: Cancer was considered a contagious disease at the middle of the 19th Century. Since bacterial etiology was the most accepted concept concerning the cause of disease, cancer also was considered a bacterial disease. In reality, it seems natural to think in such a way since certain cancers developed in certain areas or families.

In 1910, Drs. Payton and Raus of the Rockefeller Institute showed experimentally (using chickens) that a tumor can be caused by a virus. The same experiment later showed cancer in geese and turkeys caused by viruses. Such a virus theory is an extension of the previous bacterial theory of cancer.

I cannot agree with this theory. A cancerous virus is related to a decomposing cell. However, it is too hasty a conclusion to say that cancer is contagious upon finding a virus in the cancerous cell.

The concept of contagious disease is based on the theory that a "cell comes only from another cell." For example, in the case of tuberculosis let us assume that if one finds a tubercular bacillus in a diseased lung there will be two ways for the bacillus to originate. One will be the idea that this tubercular bacillus could come only from another tubercular bacillus. This last idea leads to further speculation; that is to say the tubercular bacillus resulted from infection by an outside tubercular bacillus. This is the reasoning of the contagious theory. However, no one has ever proven that the tubercular bacillus within the body came in through the respiratory tract, attached to the lung, grew, and finally caused tuberculosis. It is almost impossible to prove.

More important is that we observe the fact that a cell (especially a red blood cell) transforms to a bacteria under a bacterial-pure condition. Therefore, we can assume that there is an inverse relationship between virus, bacteria, and cell.

Virus ⟷ Bacteria ⟷ Cell

By this concept, the etiological bacteria should be considered as a decomposed cell which appears around the diseased cell. In other words, the sick, decomposed lung cell produces the tubercular bacillus. This tubercular bacillus (result) can affect another sensitive cell (cause) and promote similar destruction of tissue. In this manner, tuberculosis develops. Therefore, the tubercular bacillus is a result of the disease but in turn will cause further development of the disease.

The cancer-causing virus theory must be reconsidered from the same standpoint. Such viruses have been found even in healthy people. In short: virus, bacteria, and cell are one. Therefore, a cell can produce various vires or bacteria, the kind depending upon the condition of the cell.

In conclusion, the chemical, physical, or biological factors are secondary as the cause of cancer. The main cause of cancer exists within our body, body cell and physiological condition. These outside factors (chemical, physical, and biological) will cause cancer. However, it must be recognized that these outside factors affect inside factors such as body cells and physiological conditions. Finally, such body cells and physiological conditions are worsened resulting in the development of cancer.

How does cancer grow? Modern medicine has never doubted the concept that cancer grows by cell division. They believe the concept that cells develop only by cell division. This fixed concept is the inhibiting factor in the development of cancer research and treatment.

Drs. Shleiden and Shwann proved that cells grow by budding. Dr. Haeckell proved that cells grow from a protoplasmic state of matter which does not have cell structure, i.e., monera. O.B. Lepeshinskaya proved that the cell is generated from living matter, not from another cell. Dr. Chishima proved the same thing in a different experiment.

I have been claiming that orthodox medicine must be corrected in this "spontaneous cell generation" theory. Our "spontaneous cell generation" theory is not the widely accepted theory yet: however, nature itself will reveal its validity.

Many specimens of malignant tumors or cancers show not only typical tumor cells but also fused red blood cells which form the monera—the stage prior to the formation of the body cell structure. The end of the capillary in the tumorous tissue is open the same as that of the healthy tissue. The red blood cells that enter the gap between the tumor cells fuse together and form a "red cell monera." This monera transforms to the new body cell (which is the same kind of mother cell) by the guidance of the tumorous cell. Therefore, there is no distinction between the blood monera and the tumor cell. There is only the transient state of monera to cell.

According to the Chishima-Morishita theory, a red blood cell which is produced in the intestine wall is an immature body cell. This red blood cell transforms to the red blood monera in the gap of the tissue, and further transformation continues until the formation of the adipose tissue, muscle tissue, liver tissue, etc. is completed. The important factor influencing the transformation from monera to body cell is the biological guiding power existing in the surrounding body cells. Since the red blood cell is an immature body cell, it has no specific character. It will transform to any body cell depending on the guidance given by the surrounding cells.

The occurrence of the cell division (mitosis) in a specimen of body cancer is very difficult to recognize. However, it happens in vitro (test tube conditions). This will be explained as follows: In vitro the cell is endangered by insufficient nutrition. The cell then divides itself in order to increase its surface and efficiency of nutrification (ability to receive nutrients). In other words, cell division in vitro is a result of the cell's adaptive ability. Under physiological conditions, the cancer cell grows by the process of fusion and not by cell division.

Recently, Professor Halpern, a member of the French Academy of Medicine, stunned the cancer researchers of the world by saying that cancer cells grow not by division but by fusion. His theory is close to ours. However, it will be more perfect if he will add the concept of transformation from red blood cell to cancer cell.

Finally, I would like to add one more factor about the cause of transformation from red blood cell to cancer cell. That factor is Dr. Yanagisawa's theory concerning the acidity level of the blood, especially with respect to the decrease of Ca^{++} and the increase of Mg^{++}. *(Editor's note: further clarification was not given.)*

Chapter Four

Prevention and Cure of Cancer

The most important factor in curing cancer is the understanding of the mechanism of cancer growth. Without this knowledge, cancer is an incurable disease. Contrary to popular belief, as long as we know the cause and mechanism of cancer, cancer is not a fearful disease.

Cancer is a chronic disease, and sickness of the whole body. It may take a long time to cure, but it can be cured if the wrong medications are not applied.

There are many ways to cure cancer. For example, a simple change in the diet (from a carnivorous to vegetarian diet or from white rice to brown rice) can cure it. Cancer specialists will then say, "It wasn't cancer in the first place," because they do not know the mechanism of cancer growth. Since they do not understand the mechanism or cause of cancer, they make it an incurable disease. The term "incurable" is a mirage of modern medicine. This is especially true of the cancer, specialists. They create a public fear of cancer—cancerphobia. Such cancerphobia is an iatrogenic disease, i.e., caused by medical intervention or hospitalization.

The present cancer treatments (surgery, chemical and radiation therapies) are not suitable because they are based on a wrong concept. "Cancer can be cured if treated at an early stage" is a slogan used by modern medicine. However, this treatment is worse than the natural hygienic treatment, a power which is given us by nature.

Since modern medicine believes that a cancer cell grows by cell division, it is trying to find a chemical which will suppress such cell division. Scientists have found chemicals which will stop cell division in vitro. However, since they are very poisonous, these chemicals are harmful to our natural hygienic power when used in our body. In other words, we have to destroy our natural curing power in order to stop a so-called cancer cell division which, in reality, does not exist. This is the reason cancer is incurable. Even if we agree with the concept of these scientists, the effectiveness of such a cancer drug would be dependent upon whether the strength of the cancer cell is stronger than that of the normal body cell or not. Unfortunately, the strength of a cancer cell is usually stronger than that of a normal body cell.

As I mentioned before, the cancer cell is a kind of body cell which has been transformed from a red blood cell. This red blood cell is so immature that it can be transformed to any body cell according to the guiding power given by the surrounding body cells. When a red blood cell attaches to a cancer cell it receives strong guidance from this cell and thus transforms into another cancer cell. The power of the cancer cell is so strong that cancer cell growth is twice that of normal cell growth. Therefore, the use of chemicals to stop imagined "cancer cell division" is nonsense. Chemicals strong enough to produce an effect on cancer cells would destroy the normal body cells as well.

There are many interesting cancer treatments prescribed by Chinese and Japanese folk medicine. Pearl barley, Trapa nuts, fungus of wisteria tree, black beans, seed of burdock, etc. have been considered cancer curable agents. There must be more herbs which are effective in cancer cure. The healing power, however, is always decreased when these herbs are cultivated. Wild herbs have much stronger healing power than cultivated ones. Careful consideration of the patient's individual constitution and the stage of progress of the cancer must be given when prescribing such herbs. *(Editor's note: There are several books written about American herbs which are considered effective in cancer cure. See* Back to Eden *by Jethro Kloss.)*

General Considerations

When cancer is developing, a loss of appetite and a general anemic condition occur. From my theory, these symptoms can be explained by the following. The loss of appetite, accompanied by almost no eating, are fortunate because the physiological result of fasting causes body cells (especially cancer cells) to transform back to red blood cells. Therefore, the loss of appetite is a symptom that our natural healing power is acting.

A general anemic condition can also be very easily understood by my theory of cancer cell growth. However, modern cancer specialists advise the eating of much meat in order to increase the red blood cells. This will worsen the cancer condition. We must realize that the red blood cells made by meat are good material for the development of cancer cells when the seeds of cancer are already planted.

Cancer cells are transformed from red blood cells at a faster rate than are regular cells, thus they are not well-formed. In other words, they are clumsy and weak. Therefore, they can be transformed back to red blood cells more easily than can normal body cells. This is the reason for my previous statement about cancer not being a fearful disease.

The basic concept for a cancer cure should be the attempt to improve our natural healing power which promotes the reverse transformation of cancer cells to red blood cells.

Dr. Shelton of Texas, believing that cancer can be cured by harmony between mind and body, has had good results by promoting fasting and a fruit diet to his patients.

However, fasting as a cancer cure requires thoughtful and cautious consideration. Fasting apparently reduces cancer cells, but, at the same time, it reduces vitality. Therefore, when observing fasting as a cure, one must be aware of the difference in ratio between the reduction of cancer cells and the reduction of vitality. In fasting, care must be taken so that the reduction of vitality is not greater than the reduction of cancer cells. Therefore, I recommend fasting for cancer only by short, repeated intervals so that vitality may always be maintained.

The fruit diet would be good when the cancer is a result of eating too much meat or meat products. However, it would not be good for curing the stomach cancer of Japanese. For them, soup made of brown rice or whole grains would be better. The above mentioned herbs would also be effective.

In addition to diet and herb therapy, physical therapy should be applied. The concept for this therapy is the destruction of cancer cells through restoration of the natural healing power of our body. Static Electronic Therapy is such a treatment. The electron ion penetrates our body and stimulates the para-sympathetic nervous system. As a result, the acidity and alkalinity in our blood is balanced, and vitality of the normal cells is strengthened.

In my opinion, the three major treatments for cancer (surgery, chemical and radiation therapy) should be replaced by mental, dietetic, and physical therapy.

Prevention of Cancer

Generally speaking, the cause of cancer rests in the culmination of living conditions which have produced ill effects to the body cells. From the point of view of the cell, the cause of cancer is the malfunction of the respiratory system within the cells which results in the cell metabolism depending upon its fermenting oxidation. All living conditions which produce such a cell metabolism should be considered as the cause of cancer. Synthetic chemicals, radiations and acidification of the blood weaken the constitution of the body, and are a few of the factors which make up such living conditions. Therefore, the cure of cancer is the elimination or correction of such living conditions.

1. Live as closely as possible to nature, where water and air are clean and there is plenty of sunshine and greens.

2. Avoid commercial, processed and canned foods. Eat organically grown foods.

3. Suppress the use of synthetic chemicals. Generally speaking, all chemical drugs are poisonous. These include pesticides, preservatives, sterilization drugs, disinfectants, antibiotics and chemical condiments.

4. Work and exercise well. This helps to improve any malfunctioning of the respiratory function of the cells. It will result in good sleep, appetite and bowel movement.

5. Avoid mental stress by studying the teachings of ancient sages. These include such teachings as the Unique Principle by George Ohsawa and Chinese or Indian philosophy.

How to Observe
a Macrobiotic Diet

There are two basic ways to attain health, freedom, and happiness in this life: (1) by unveiling our Supreme Judgment (awareness of Absolute Truth), and (2) by applying unifying principle (yin-yang) to our selection and preparation of mainly locally grown whole foods.

Although seemingly different ways, these two actions are deeply related because our brain cells are the vehicles of our Judgment (Supreme), and the conditions of our brain cells are affected by our judgment (yin-yang) in selecting and preparing the foods we eat.

Many people therefore wonder: "I must eat well in order to raise my judgment and thereby unveil my Judgment, but how can I eat well when my judgment is so low?" The most common error at this point is paranoia: "I will eat virtually nothing but grains until I am healthy, at which point my judgment will be very high, and my Judgment will be unveiled." Such a rigid way of eating does have one advantage—it makes such a big change in one's body and brain, so quickly, that one is unlikely ever again to doubt the importance of food. But if it is persisted in for more than a week or so, it will be harmful.

It is true that health, freedom and happiness are more likely to come to those who base their diet mainly on foods that are relatively near the middle of the yin-yang spectrum, and that grains are therefore the most healthful principal foods for man in most climatic zones. But since most of us have been eating so far out on both sides of the spectrum, very extreme reactions will occur if we suddenly switch to and try to maintain a way of eating which includes a very limited variety of foods. Those of us who have taken more than very small amounts of meat, sugar or (especially) drugs have reduced to a very great extent our ability to produce (transmute from such a limited diet all (or even most) of the nutrients we need in order to establish and maintain our physical and mental health.

We often forget that most of us have developed our poor health over a period of several years, and that it will also therefore, take us time to recover our strength, vitality and clarity of judgment. And that's why it's important to establish a way of eating that can be maintained for more than a few days or weeks. And a strict, rigid and extremely limited diet is not a way of eating that is conducive to being maintained. It forces the body to attempt to revamp its entire digestive apparatus almost overnight, violently shocks our nervous systems, abruptly releases stored-up toxins into our bloodstreams, and results in many nutritional deficiencies—thus leading us to become helplessly attracted to the extremes of eating which caused our poor health and low judgment in the first place.

For those of us who have drastically reduced our transmuting ability, vegetables (cooked and raw), beans, seaweeds, nuts, fruits, fish and dairy products are not luxuries; they are necessities.

Another approach, which is more effective than the fanatical one described above, is to imitate macrobiotic eating by observing and trying to practice the eating habits of those who have been trying to eat macrobiotically for several months or years. But this approach also has a disadvantage—which is that there are many people who, even after several years of what they consider to be macrobiotic eating, have still attained neither health, freedom nor happiness.

Why? Because they have not yet understood the principle (yin-yang) behind macrobiotic eating. For example, if a person living in a hot climate were to maintain an eating pattern consisting of about 70% grains; 15% cooked vegetables, beans and seaweeds; 10% fish and/or dairy products; 5% raw vegetables; and little or no nuts or fruits, that person would not be eating macrobiotically (he would be eating much too yang). Yet such an eating pattern would be quite suitable for the average person living in a cold climate. If we do not adapt our eating to our climate, age, sex, amount and type of activity, and previous eating habits, we are not eating macrobiotically. In short, imitation can be very useful—especially to those who are in the first few days or weeks of trying to eat macrobiotically—but in the long run, it too is not the way to success.

The following are our suggestions for those who want to establish their health as quickly as possible and maintain it:

1. Try, as much as possible, to eat mainly locally grown (from within about 500 miles) whole foods. Avoid all derivatives, such as vitamin pills, wheat germ, white rice, juices (unless you also eat the rest of the fruit or vegetable) and all synthetic chemicals.

2. Remember that the amount of salt (unrefined "crude" is best) we use strongly influences our judgment in selecting and preparing the rest of our diet. If in doubt, use less—particularly when you become strongly attracted to sugar or other extremely yin foods. Some general guidelines on salt are that babies and the elderly need less than others; men need more than women; those who are very active physically need more; and we all need less in hot weather than in cold.

3. Avoid elaborate and/or painfully difficult rules of eating; instead, let your desires help you to discover and adapt to constantly changing needs.

4. Study the unifying principle in terms of your own actions and thinking; be objective—don't take anybody's advice blindly.

About the Author

Dr. Keiichi Morishita is one of the few modern scientists who have confirmed George Ohsawa's conclusion that blood is made from food in the intestines of the normally functioning human organism.

A man who lives his beliefs, Dr. Morishita ranks high in the eyes of the medical profession, yet is a practicing macrobiotic, and is also remarkable in that he is interested not only in his chosen field of medical science, but also in astronomy, philosophy and the macroscopic origins of life.

Majoring in blood physiology, Dr. Morishita did his undergraduate work in Tokyo Medical University where he graduated in 1930. In 1935, he received his Doctor of Medicine Degree and was later appointed Assistant Professor of Physiology at the same university. In 1937, he taught at the Dental School of the University and, in 1944, became Technical Chief for the Tokyo Red Cross Blood Center. Dr. Morishita is presently a member of the Physiology Association of Japan, president of the Life Sciences Association, and vice-president of the New Blood Association.

Author of countless research papers for the academic community, Dr. Morishita has also written several books for the general public including:

> *The Origin of the Blood Cell*
> *Foundations of Physiology*
> *The Degradation of Life*
> *Blood and Cancer*

These four books are presently available only in Japanese. *The Hidden Truth of Cancer* has been translated here by Herman Aihara, a noted macrobiotic teacher and formerly leader of the George Ohsawa Macrobiotic Foundation.

Printed in Great Britain
by Amazon

24627329R00030